ORNISH DIET COOKBOOK

Guide To Reversing Heart Disease And Losing Weight with Ornish diet

Alex Kava

Copyright

Table of Contents

Introduction

Once upon a time in a quiet suburban neighborhood, there lived a woman named Sarah who had been struggling with her health for years. She had tried countless diets, exercise programs, and fad solutions, but nothing seemed to work. Her doctor had recently informed her that she needed to make significant changes to her lifestyle to combat her rising cholesterol levels and prevent heart disease. Sarah was feeling overwhelmed and hopeless until one day, while browsing the local library, she stumbled upon a book with a promising title: **"The Ornish Diet Cookbook."**

Intrigued, Sarah picked up the book and began to flip through its pages. She was immediately struck by the amazing Chapter of the book, wholesome dishes that filled the pages. The recipes seemed both delicious and nourishing, and the thought of a diet that could potentially reverse her health issues ignited a spark of hope within her.

Without hesitation, Sarah checked out the book and headed home. Over the next few days, she immersed herself in its pages, absorbing the principles of the Ornish Diet. The emphasis on plant-based foods, low-fat ingredients, and mindful eating resonated with her. She realized that this could be the answer she had been searching for all along.

With newfound determination, Sarah started experimenting with the recipes in the cookbook. She began incorporating more fruits, vegetables, grains, and legumes into her meals, replacing high-fat ingredients with healthier alternatives. Each dish she prepared was a culinary adventure, and she was amazed by how tasty and satisfying the food was.

As the weeks went by, Sarah's health began to transform. Her energy levels increased, and she found herself shedding excess weight. Most importantly, her cholesterol levels started to drop, and her doctor was pleasantly surprised by the positive changes. Sarah's confidence grew with each passing day, and she felt a renewed sense of purpose.

But it wasn't just about the physical changes. Sarah also noticed an improvement in her emotional well-being. The act of preparing and savoring each meal mindfully brought her a sense of peace and contentment she had never experienced before. She realized that the Ornish Diet wasn't just about what she ate; it was about how she lived her life.

Over time, Sarah's success with the **Ornish Diet Cookbook** became an inspiration to her friends and family. They witnessed her transformation and wanted to join her on this journey to better health. Together, they explored the joys of cooking and sharing nutritious, flavorful meals.

Sarah's story serves as a reminder that sometimes, the answer to our health challenges can be found within the pages of a book. **The Ornish Diet Cookbook** not only helped her regain her health but also brought a newfound love for food and a deep appreciation for the power of mindful eating into her life. It was a story of transformation, hope, and the incredible potential that lies within a simple book title.

Chapter 1: Understanding the Ornish Diet

The Ornish Diet, developed by Dr. Dean Ornish, is a renowned and scientifically-backed approach to improving heart health and overall well-being. This dietary plan is part of a comprehensive lifestyle program that emphasizes not only what you eat but also how you live. Dr. Ornish's work has been instrumental in demonstrating the power of lifestyle changes in preventing and even reversing heart disease.

The Ornish Diet is often associated with reversing heart disease, but its principles can also promote weight loss, reduce the risk of other chronic diseases, and enhance overall vitality. To fully grasp the essence of the Ornish Diet, it's important to delve into its key components and underlying philosophy:

1. Low-Fat, Plant-Based Nutrition: At the core of the Ornish Diet is a focus on whole, plant-based foods. This means consuming a variety of fruits, vegetables, whole grains, legumes, and nuts while minimizing or eliminating animal products. The diet is extremely low in fat, particularly saturated fat, which is a major contributor to heart disease.

2. Complex Carbohydrates: The diet encourages the consumption of complex carbohydrates, such as whole grains and starchy vegetables. These provide sustained energy and are rich in fiber, which aids in digestion and helps control blood sugar levels.

3. Limited Refined Sugar and Simple Carbs: To maintain stable blood sugar levels and promote overall health, the Ornish Diet recommends avoiding or severely limiting foods and beverages high in refined sugars and simple carbohydrates.

4. Minimal Fat Intake: The diet restricts the intake of fats to around 10% of total daily calories. This includes minimizing the use of oils, especially those high in saturated fats, like palm and coconut oil. Instead, small amounts of unsaturated fats, like those found in avocados and nuts, are encouraged.

5. Portion Control: The Ornish Diet emphasizes portion control to manage calorie intake effectively. Eating mindfully and paying attention to hunger and fullness cues are crucial components.

6. Regular Physical Activity: Alongside dietary changes, regular physical activity is an integral part of the Ornish program. Exercise helps improve cardiovascular health, aids in weight management, and boosts overall well-being.

7. Stress Reduction: Managing stress is another pillar of the Ornish program. Techniques such as yoga, meditation, and mindfulness are promoted to reduce stress, which can contribute to heart disease.

8. Social Support: Dr. Ornish emphasizes the importance of a supportive social network. Sharing your journey with others who have similar goals can provide motivation and accountability.

9. Moderate Alcohol Consumption: While alcohol can have some heart benefits in moderation, the Ornish Diet suggests limiting alcohol intake.

10. No Smoking: Smoking cessation is vital in the Ornish program, as smoking is a major risk factor for heart disease.

It's important to note that the Ornish Diet is not just a diet but a comprehensive lifestyle program. Dr. Ornish's research has shown that this holistic approach can lead to remarkable improvements in heart health, including the reversal of atherosclerosis (the narrowing of arteries), reduced cholesterol levels, and improved blood pressure.

Moreover, the Ornish Diet isn't just about treating existing heart disease; it's also a preventive strategy. By adopting these principles, individuals can reduce their risk of developing heart disease and other chronic illnesses.

The Ornish Diet offers a holistic approach to heart health and overall well-being. It combines a low-fat, plant-based diet with regular exercise, stress management, and social support. Understanding the Ornish Diet means recognizing the interconnectedness of lifestyle choices and their profound impact on health, making it a valuable resource for those seeking to improve their cardiovascular health and overall quality of life.

Origins and Principles of the Ornish Diet

The Ornish Diet, developed by Dr. Dean Ornish, has its roots in extensive research on lifestyle and its impact on heart health. Dr. Ornish's pioneering work has not only reshaped our understanding of cardiovascular disease but has also provided a clear path to prevention and even reversal of this deadly condition. Let's delve into the origins and key principles that underpin the Ornish Diet.

Origins of the Ornish Diet:

Dr. Dean Ornish, a cardiologist and researcher, began his groundbreaking work in the early 1990s. His studies challenged conventional wisdom about heart disease, which often focused primarily on medications and invasive procedures. Instead, Dr. Ornish sought to explore the potential of comprehensive lifestyle changes to address heart disease at its core.

One of the most notable studies that brought the Ornish Diet to the forefront was the Lifestyle Heart Trial, published in 1990. In this trial, Dr. Ornish and his team demonstrated that lifestyle modifications, including a low-fat, plant-based diet, regular exercise, stress reduction, and social support, could not only halt the progression of coronary artery disease but also reverse it. This landmark research laid the foundation for the Ornish Diet and his broader program for heart health.

Key Principles of the Ornish Diet:

1. Low-Fat, Plant-Based Nutrition: The cornerstone of the Ornish Diet is a diet that is primarily plant-based. It promotes the consumption of whole foods, such as fruits, vegetables, whole grains, legumes, and nuts. This plant-centric approach is naturally low in fat, particularly saturated fat, which is a major contributor to the development of atherosclerosis (the hardening and narrowing of arteries).

2. Emphasis on Complex Carbohydrates: The diet encourages the intake of complex carbohydrates found in whole grains, which provide a steady source of energy and are rich in fiber, vitamins, and minerals. These carbohydrates help stabilize blood sugar levels and promote long-term health.

3. Minimal Saturated and Trans Fats: The Ornish Diet recommends strict limitations on saturated and trans fats, which are commonly found in animal products and processed foods. These fats are known to raise cholesterol levels and contribute to heart disease.

4. Limited Sugar and Refined Carbohydrates: To maintain optimal blood sugar control and overall health, the diet advises reducing the consumption of refined sugars and simple carbohydrates, such as those found in sugary snacks and beverages.

5. Portion Control: Understanding portion sizes is key to calorie management. The Ornish Diet encourages mindful eating and paying attention to hunger and fullness cues.

6. Moderate Protein: While the diet is primarily plant-based, it does include moderate amounts of protein from sources like beans, lentils, and soy products. This can help meet protein requirements without relying heavily on animal products.

7. Stress Reduction: Stress is a significant risk factor for heart disease. The Ornish program incorporates stress management techniques like yoga, meditation, and mindfulness to reduce emotional and psychological stress.

8. Regular Physical Activity: Exercise is a fundamental component of the Ornish Diet. Engaging in regular physical activity not only supports weight management but also contributes to overall cardiovascular health.

9. Social Support: Building a supportive social network is encouraged in the Ornish program. Sharing experiences, challenges, and successes with others who have similar health goals can provide motivation and accountability.

10. No Smoking: Smoking cessation is a non-negotiable aspect of the Ornish program. Smoking is a potent risk factor for heart disease, and quitting is crucial for cardiovascular health.

The Ornish Diet is a comprehensive lifestyle program that extends beyond just dietary guidelines. It emphasizes the interplay between nutrition, exercise, stress management, and social support in achieving optimal heart health. This holistic approach has not only been instrumental in treating and preventing heart disease but has also inspired a broader understanding of how lifestyle choices can profoundly impact our overall well-being.

Benefits for Heart Health and Weight Loss

The Ornish Diet is not only renowned for its holistic approach to heart health but also for its potential to aid in weight loss and overall well-being. This dietary plan, designed by Dr. Dean Ornish, offers a range of benefits that extend beyond cardiovascular health. Let's explore how the Ornish Diet can positively impact heart health and support weight loss efforts.

Benefits for Heart Health:

1. Reversal of Heart Disease: One of the most striking benefits of the Ornish Diet is its potential to reverse coronary artery disease. Dr. Ornish's pioneering research has demonstrated that comprehensive lifestyle changes, including adherence to this diet, can lead to the regression of atherosclerosis—the narrowing of arteries due to plaque buildup. This means that, in some cases, individuals can improve their heart health to the point where arteries become less blocked, reducing the risk of heart attacks.

2. Reduced Cholesterol Levels: The diet's emphasis on low-fat, plant-based foods, and the avoidance of saturated and trans fats helps lower cholesterol levels in the blood. Elevated cholesterol is a key risk factor for heart disease, and the Ornish Diet can contribute to substantial reductions in both LDL (bad) cholesterol and total cholesterol.

3. Better Blood Pressure Control: By incorporating whole, unprocessed foods and reducing sodium intake, the Ornish Diet can have a positive impact on blood pressure. Lowering blood pressure is crucial for reducing the risk of hypertension and related heart problems.

4. Improved Blood Sugar Control: The diet's focus on complex carbohydrates and low sugar intake helps stabilize blood sugar levels, which is vital for individuals with diabetes or those at risk of developing the condition. Maintaining healthy blood sugar levels can reduce the risk of heart disease.

5. Weight Management: While weight loss is not the primary goal of the Ornish Diet, many individuals do experience weight loss as a natural outcome of the diet's principles. The emphasis on whole, fiber-rich foods and portion control can support gradual and sustainable weight reduction.

Benefits for Weight Loss:

1. Whole, Nutrient-Dense Foods: The Ornish Diet promotes the consumption of nutrient-dense, whole foods that are naturally low in calories. This includes fruits, vegetables, whole grains, and legumes, which can help individuals feel satisfied while managing their calorie intake.

2. Reduced Saturated Fat: By minimizing or eliminating animal products and high-fat foods, the diet reduces saturated fat consumption, which is linked to weight gain. Lowering saturated fat intake can contribute to better weight control.

3. Portion Control: The Ornish Diet encourages mindful eating and portion control, which are essential for managing calorie intake and preventing overeating.

4. Balanced Macronutrients: The diet provides a balanced distribution of macronutrients, including carbohydrates, protein, and healthy fats. This balance can help maintain energy levels and prevent extreme fluctuations in blood sugar that can trigger cravings.

5. Sustainable Lifestyle: The Ornish Diet isn't a crash diet but a sustainable lifestyle. Its focus on overall well-being and the inclusion of stress management and social support can contribute to long-term weight management success.

6. Reduction in Emotional Eating: Stress reduction techniques, such as meditation and yoga, are integral to the Ornish program. These practices can help individuals better manage emotional eating, a common obstacle to weight loss.

It's important to note that the Ornish Diet may not be suitable for everyone, and individual results can vary. Consulting with a healthcare provider or a registered dietitian is advisable before starting any new diet or lifestyle program, especially if you have specific medical conditions or dietary restrictions.

The Ornish Diet offers a multifaceted approach to health. Its focus on plant-based, low-fat nutrition, combined with stress management and exercise, can significantly improve heart health and support weight loss. By adopting these principles, individuals can enhance their overall well-being and reduce their risk of heart disease while working toward achieving and maintaining a healthy weight.

Chapter 2: Getting Started with the Ornish Diet

The Ornish Diet, developed by Dr. Dean Ornish, is a renowned and scientifically-proven approach to improving your health and well-being through dietary choices and lifestyle changes. It is well-known for its focus on reversing heart disease and promoting overall health. If you're looking to adopt a heart-healthy, plant-based diet and make positive changes in your life, getting started with the Ornish Diet is a great step in the right direction.

Understanding the Ornish Diet

The Ornish Diet is primarily a plant-based diet that emphasizes whole foods and limits the consumption of animal products, saturated fats, and processed foods. It is designed to reduce the risk of heart disease and other chronic conditions by promoting heart-healthy eating patterns and lifestyle modifications. Here are some key principles to help you understand the Ornish Diet:

1. Plant-Centric Approach:

- Focus on consuming a wide variety of colorful fruits and vegetables. These are rich in essential vitamins, minerals, and antioxidants that promote overall health.

- Include whole grains like brown rice, quinoa, and whole wheat bread in your meals.

- Legumes, such as beans, lentils, and chickpeas, are excellent sources of protein and fiber and should be a staple in your diet.

2. Minimal Animal Products:

- The Ornish Diet encourages the consumption of low-fat or fat-free dairy products, like yogurt and milk. However, these should be limited.

- Poultry and fish can be included in moderation but should be prepared without skin and visible fat.

- Red meat, especially processed and high-fat cuts, is discouraged or should be consumed very sparingly.

3. Healthy Fats:

- Choose heart-healthy fats such as avocados, nuts, and seeds in moderation.

- Minimize or eliminate saturated and trans fats, often found in fried and processed foods.

4. Portion Control:

- Be mindful of portion sizes to avoid overeating. Practice portion control to maintain a healthy weight and promote heart health.

5. Lifestyle Changes:

- In addition to dietary changes, the Ornish Diet emphasizes stress management techniques, regular exercise, and social support as vital components of a heart-healthy lifestyle.

Getting Started

Embarking on the Ornish Diet involves gradual changes to your eating habits and lifestyle. Here are some steps to help you get started:

1. Consult a Healthcare Professional:

- Before making any significant dietary changes, it's advisable to consult a healthcare professional, especially if you have any underlying medical conditions or concerns.

2. Set Realistic Goals:

- Define your goals for adopting the Ornish Diet. Whether it's reducing cholesterol levels, losing weight, or improving overall health, having clear objectives will help you stay motivated.

3. Educate Yourself:

- Learn about the principles of the Ornish Diet by reading books, articles, and reputable sources. Understanding why certain foods are included and others are restricted can make the transition easier.

4. Start Slowly:

- Transitioning to a new way of eating can be challenging. Begin by incorporating more plant-based foods into your diet gradually. Replace one or two animal-based meals per week with plant-based alternatives.

5. Plan Your Meals:

- Create a meal plan that includes a variety of fruits, vegetables, whole grains, and legumes. Experiment with different recipes to keep your meals interesting and delicious.

6. Monitor Progress:

- Keep track of your dietary choices and their impact on your health. Regularly check your cholesterol levels, blood pressure, and weight to gauge your progress.

7. Engage in Physical Activity:

- Incorporate regular exercise into your routine. Aim for at least 150 minutes of moderate-intensity aerobic activity per week, as recommended by health experts.

8. Seek Support:

- Consider joining a support group or finding a buddy who shares your dietary goals. Having a support system can help you stay on track and motivated.

Remember that the Ornish Diet is not just a short-term solution but a sustainable way of living that can lead to long-lasting health benefits. By making these gradual changes and embracing a plant-based, heart-healthy lifestyle, you can significantly improve your overall well-being and reduce the risk of chronic diseases.

Preparing Your Kitchen

Embarking on a new dietary journey can be both exciting and challenging. The Ornish Diet, developed by Dr. Dean Ornish, is a well-regarded and scientifically-backed approach to improving your overall health and well-being through diet and lifestyle changes. Before diving into the specifics of meal planning and recipes, it's essential to set the stage by preparing your kitchen. A well-organized and stocked kitchen can make a significant difference in your success with the Ornish Diet. In this guide, we'll walk you through the steps to get your kitchen ready for this heart-healthy and transformative eating plan.

1. Clear Out the Clutter

Before you start stocking your kitchen with Ornish-approved foods, take some time to declutter and organize your space. This not only makes meal preparation more efficient but also helps you stay focused on your dietary goals. Here's what to do:

- **Clean Out Your Pantry:** Go through your pantry and refrigerator to identify and remove any items that don't align with the Ornish Diet principles. This includes processed foods, sugary snacks, and high-fat dairy products.

- **Check Expiry Dates:** Discard expired or stale items to make room for fresh, wholesome ingredients.

- **Organize Your Shelves:** Arrange your pantry and refrigerator so that healthier options are at eye level and easily accessible. This will help you make better choices when you're hungry.

2. Stock Up on Essentials

Now that you've cleared out the unhealthy options, it's time to stock your kitchen with the essentials of the Ornish Diet. The core principles of this diet include:

- **High-fiber foods:** Whole grains like brown rice, quinoa, and whole wheat pasta are staples. Include legumes like lentils, beans, and chickpeas for added fiber and protein.

- **Fruits and Vegetables:** Load up on a variety of colorful fruits and vegetables, as they form the foundation of this diet. Fresh, frozen, or canned (with no added salt or sugar) options are all suitable choices.

- **Lean Proteins:** Opt for plant-based proteins such as tofu, tempeh, and edamame. If you choose animal proteins, go for skinless poultry, fish (especially fatty fish like salmon), and occasional servings of lean cuts of meat.

- **Healthy Fats:** Incorporate sources of healthy fats like avocados, nuts, seeds, and olive oil, but use them sparingly.

- **Low-Fat Dairy (optional):** If you consume dairy, choose low-fat or fat-free options. Otherwise, consider dairy alternatives like almond milk or soy yogurt.

- **Herbs and Spices:** Ditch the salt and opt for a variety of herbs and spices to flavor your dishes. This reduces sodium intake while enhancing the taste of your meals.

3. Equip Your Kitchen

Having the right tools and equipment in your kitchen can make meal preparation easier and more enjoyable. Consider investing in:

- **A Sharp Knife Set:** Quality knives make chopping vegetables and fruits a breeze.

- Pots and Pans: Non-stick cookware helps reduce the need for excessive cooking oil.

- Steamer Basket: This handy tool makes steaming vegetables a quick and healthy cooking option.

- Blender or Food Processor: These appliances are excellent for creating smoothies, soups, and sauces.

- Measuring Cups and Spoons: Accurate measurements are essential when following specific recipes.

- Storage Containers: Prepare and store healthy meals and snacks for convenient on-the-go options.

4. Plan Your Meals

Meal planning is crucial when following the Ornish Diet. Before you go grocery shopping, sit down and plan your meals for the week. Create a shopping list based on your menu to ensure you only purchase what you need, reducing food waste and the temptation to buy unhealthy items.

5. Read Labels Carefully

When shopping for packaged foods, take the time to read nutrition labels. Look for products that are low in saturated fats, trans fats, sodium, and added sugars. The Ornish Diet encourages whole, minimally processed foods, so try to limit your intake of processed items as much as possible.

6. Stay Informed

Lastly, educate yourself about the Ornish Diet's principles and guidelines. Understand the types of foods you should focus on and those you should avoid. Being well-informed will help you make healthier choices when shopping and cooking.

preparing your kitchen for the Ornish Diet is an essential first step in your journey to better health. By decluttering, stocking up on essentials, equipping your kitchen with the right tools, and planning your meals, you'll set yourself up for success as you embark on this heart-healthy eating plan. Remember that the Ornish Diet is not just about what you eat but also about adopting a holistic approach to wellness that includes stress management, exercise, and social support. With dedication and preparation, you can make positive changes that will benefit your overall health and well-being.

Stocking Ornish-Friendly Ingredients

Now that you've prepared your kitchen by decluttering, organizing, and equipping it for success on the Ornish Diet, it's time to focus on stocking it with Ornish-friendly ingredients. The Ornish Diet places a strong emphasis on whole, plant-based foods and limits the intake of animal products and high-fat options. In this guide, we'll help you identify the essential ingredients you should have on hand to create delicious, heart-healthy meals.

1. Whole Grains

Whole grains are the foundation of the Ornish Diet. They provide essential fiber, vitamins, and minerals while promoting a sense of fullness. Stock up on:

- **Brown Rice:** Versatile and nutrient-rich, brown rice is a staple in many Ornish Diet recipes.

- **Quinoa:** A complete protein source, quinoa is an excellent choice for salads and side dishes.

- **Whole Wheat Pasta:** Choose whole wheat pasta over refined options for added fiber.

- **Oats:** Perfect for oatmeal, smoothies, and baking.

- **Whole Wheat Bread:** Look for whole wheat or whole grain bread with minimal added sugar.

2. Fruits and Vegetables

Colorful fruits and vegetables are rich in antioxidants, vitamins, and minerals, making them a crucial component of the Ornish Diet. Fresh, frozen, or canned (with no added sugar or salt) are all good choices. Stock your kitchen with a variety of:

- **Leafy Greens:** Spinach, kale, and Swiss chard are packed with nutrients.

- **Berries:** Blueberries, strawberries, and raspberries are low in calories and high in antioxidants.

- **Citrus Fruits:** Oranges, grapefruits, and lemons add a zesty, tangy flavor.

- **Cruciferous Vegetables:** Broccoli, cauliflower, and Brussels sprouts offer cancer-fighting properties.

- **Root Vegetables:** Sweet potatoes and carrots provide essential vitamins and fiber.

- **Tomatoes:** Fresh tomatoes or canned tomatoes without added salt can be used in sauces and soups.

3. Legumes

Legumes are an excellent source of plant-based protein and fiber. They're versatile and can be used in various dishes. Stock up on:

- **Lentils:** Quick-cooking and full of protein, lentils are perfect for soups and stews.

- **Chickpeas:** Great for making hummus, salads, and curry dishes.

- **Black Beans:** Use in burritos, salads, or as a meat substitute in recipes.

- **Kidney Beans:** Ideal for chili and bean-based dishes.

4. Plant-Based Proteins

To reduce your intake of animal products, incorporate plant-based protein sources into your diet:

- **Tofu:** A versatile protein that takes on the flavors of the dishes you prepare.

- **Tempeh:** A fermented soy product that adds a nutty flavor to recipes.

- **Edamame:** Young soybeans can be steamed and seasoned for a healthy snack.

- **Seitan:** Made from wheat gluten, seitan is an excellent meat substitute.

5. Lean Proteins (Optional)

If you choose to include animal products, opt for lean sources:

- **Skinless Poultry:** Chicken and turkey breast are lower in saturated fat.

- **Fish:** Fatty fish like salmon and trout are rich in omega-3 fatty acids.

6. Healthy Fats

While the Ornish Diet is low in fat, it does include small amounts of healthy fats:

- **Avocado:** Rich in monounsaturated fats and perfect for salads and spreads.

- **Nuts and Seeds:** Almonds, walnuts, flaxseeds, and chia seeds are excellent choices in moderation.

- **Olive Oil:** Use extra-virgin olive oil sparingly for cooking or dressing salads.

7. Herbs and Spices

Instead of relying on salt and high-fat condiments, flavor your dishes with herbs and spices like:

- **Basil:** Fresh or dried basil adds a fragrant note to many recipes.

- **Cumin:** Adds warmth and depth to dishes like chili and curries.

- **Turmeric:** Known for its anti-inflammatory properties, turmeric is a staple in Indian cuisine.

- **Cinnamon:** A versatile spice for both sweet and savory dishes.

8. Low-Fat Dairy (Optional)

If you choose to include dairy, opt for low-fat or fat-free options:

- **Greek Yogurt:** High in protein and versatile for breakfast or as a topping.

- **Skim Milk:** A lower-fat alternative for coffee and cereal.

- **Low-Fat Cheese:** Use sparingly for added flavor in recipes.

By stocking your kitchen with these Ornish-friendly ingredients, you'll be well-prepared to create delicious, heart-healthy meals that align with the principles of the Ornish Diet. Remember to stay creative in the kitchen, experiment with different combinations of these ingredients, and enjoy the journey towards better health and well-being.

Meal Planning Tips

Meal planning is a crucial component of successfully adopting the Ornish Diet. Proper planning ensures that you have a variety of heart-healthy meals readily available, making it easier to stick to the principles of this dietary approach. Here are some valuable meal planning tips to help you get started on the Ornish Diet:

1. Set Clear Goals

Before you begin meal planning, establish your specific health goals. Are you looking to lower your cholesterol, manage your weight, or improve your overall well-being? Understanding your objectives will guide your food choices and portion sizes.

2. Create a Weekly Meal Schedule

Planning your meals for the week can save you time, money, and stress. Designate a specific time each week to sit down and plan your menu. Consider your schedule, daily activities, and any special occasions or events that might affect your dietary choices.

3. Balance Your Meals

A balanced Ornish Diet meal typically includes:

- **Vegetables:** Make vegetables the star of your plate. Aim to fill half your plate with colorful, non-starchy veggies.

- **Whole Grains:** Incorporate whole grains like brown rice, quinoa, or whole wheat pasta to provide energy and fiber.

- **Legumes:** Include beans, lentils, or chickpeas for plant-based protein.

- **Lean Proteins (optional):** If you choose animal proteins, keep portions small and opt for lean cuts.

- **Healthy Fats:** Add sources of healthy fats like avocado, nuts, and seeds in moderation.

4. Plan for Snacks

Healthy snacks can help you maintain your energy levels throughout the day and prevent overeating during meals. Stock your kitchen with Ornish-approved snacks like fresh fruit, raw vegetables with hummus, or a small serving of unsalted nuts.

5. Batch Cooking

Save time by preparing larger quantities of certain dishes and freezing portions for later use. For example, cook a big batch of vegetable soup, chili, or grain-based salads that can be portioned and frozen for quick, convenient meals.

6. Embrace Leftovers

Don't underestimate the power of leftovers. When preparing dinner, make extra portions to enjoy for lunch the next day. This reduces food waste and ensures you have a nutritious meal readily available.

7. Incorporate Variety

Eating the same foods day in and day out can lead to boredom and make it challenging to stick to your diet. Experiment with different vegetables, grains, and protein sources to keep your meals exciting and flavorful.

8. Read Labels

When shopping for packaged foods, carefully read the labels to ensure they meet the Ornish Diet guidelines. Look for products low in saturated fats, trans fats, sodium, and added sugars. Avoid items with excessive processing or artificial ingredients.

9. Plan for Special Occasions

Social events and dining out can pose challenges to your meal plan. Plan ahead by checking restaurant menus for heart-healthy options or offer to bring a dish to gatherings that align with your dietary goals.

10. Stay Hydrated

Proper hydration is essential for overall health. Drink plenty of water throughout the day. You can also enjoy herbal teas or infused water for added variety.

11. Monitor Portions

Even when eating healthily, portion control is vital for managing your calorie intake. Invest in measuring cups and a food scale to accurately portion your meals.

12. Be Flexible

Remember that life can be unpredictable, and there may be days when your meal plan doesn't go as expected. Don't be too hard on yourself; flexibility is key to long-term success. Make the best choices you can in any given situation.

13. Seek Support

Consider joining a support group or finding a diet buddy who shares your commitment to the Ornish Diet. Having someone to discuss challenges and successes with can be incredibly motivating.

Meal planning on the Ornish Diet may require some initial effort, but the long-term benefits to your health and well-being are well worth it. By setting clear goals, creating a meal schedule, balancing your meals, and incorporating these tips into your routine, you'll be well-prepared to make sustainable and heart-healthy dietary choices.

Chapter 3: Delicious Breakfasts

Breakfast, often hailed as the most important meal of the day, is a delightful moment to kickstart your morning with a burst of energy and flavor. Whether you're a fan of sweet or savory, traditional or adventurous, there's a breakfast option for every palate. From classic favorites to global inspirations, let's embark on a culinary journey exploring the world of delicious breakfasts.

1. Classic American Breakfast: Few things beat the comforting aroma of crispy bacon, fluffy pancakes, and perfectly scrambled eggs. Add a dollop of maple syrup, a side of fresh fruit, and a steaming cup of coffee, and you have a quintessential American breakfast that never goes out of style.

2. Continental Elegance: If you prefer a touch of European sophistication in your morning meal, consider a continental breakfast. Croissants, pain au chocolat, and buttery brioche accompanied by rich coffee or freshly squeezed orange juice transport you to a Parisian café.

3. Mexican Fiesta: Spice up your morning with a Mexican-inspired breakfast. Huevos Rancheros, breakfast burritos, or chilaquiles offer a burst of flavors with ingredients like salsa, avocados, and black beans. Don't forget the hot sauce for that extra kick.

4. Healthy Start: For those looking for a healthier option, a Greek yogurt parfait topped with granola and fresh berries is a delicious choice. It provides a satisfying blend of protein and fiber to keep you energized throughout the day.

5. Asian Fusion: Try a breakfast bowl inspired by Asian cuisine. A steaming bowl of miso soup, paired with rice, grilled fish, and pickled vegetables, offers a unique and savory way to begin your day.

6. Oatmeal Variations: Oatmeal lovers can experiment with various toppings like honey, nuts, fruits, and spices to create their signature bowls. Overnight oats and steel-cut oatmeal are excellent choices for a wholesome breakfast.

7. Vegan Delights: For plant-based eaters, there are plenty of scrumptious options. Avocado toast with cherry tomatoes and a sprinkle of nutritional yeast or a tofu scramble with veggies are both flavorful and cruelty-free choices.

8. South Indian Sensation: Dosa, idli, or upma, South Indian breakfasts are a symphony of flavors. Accompanied by coconut chutney, sambar, or a tangy tomato relish, they provide a burst of taste that's hard to resist.

9. Mediterranean Magic: A Mediterranean breakfast often includes fresh olives, feta cheese, tomatoes, and cucumbers, served with warm pita bread. Drizzle some olive oil and sprinkle za'atar seasoning for an authentic touch.

10. Global Influences: In today's interconnected world, breakfasts have taken on influences from all corners of the globe. You can find Korean kimchi toast, Japanese tamago sushi, or Middle Eastern shakshuka in trendy breakfast spots around the world.

A delicious breakfast not only satisfies your taste buds but also provides the necessary nutrients to fuel your body for the day ahead. Whether you prefer a quick and simple meal or a leisurely brunch spread, the choices are endless. So, why not start your day with a culinary adventure and make breakfast a celebration of flavors and cultures? Your taste buds will thank you, and you'll be ready to conquer the day with a smile.

Nutrient-Packed Smoothies

In the quest for a convenient, healthy, and delicious breakfast option, nutrient-packed smoothies have emerged as a popular choice. These blended concoctions offer a delightful way to kickstart your day with a burst of vitamins, minerals, fiber, and essential nutrients. Whether you're in a rush or prefer a leisurely morning routine, smoothies are versatile and easily customizable to suit your taste and nutritional needs. Let's dive into the world of delicious breakfast smoothies and explore the endless possibilities.

The Smoothie Basics

A typical breakfast smoothie usually consists of a few key components:

1. Base: This is the liquid component that forms the foundation of your smoothie. Common choices include almond milk, coconut water, yogurt, or even plain water.

2. Fruits and Vegetables: These provide the flavor, natural sweetness, and a dose of essential vitamins and minerals. Berries, bananas, spinach, kale, and avocados are popular choices.

3. Protein: Adding protein to your smoothie helps keep you full and provides sustained energy throughout the morning. You can opt for protein powder, Greek yogurt, or nut butter.

4. Fiber: Fiber-rich ingredients like oats, chia seeds, or flaxseed not only promote digestive health but also contribute to the smoothie's texture and satiety.

5. Extras: Get creative with superfoods and extras such as spirulina, matcha, honey, or spices like cinnamon and ginger to enhance both flavor and nutritional value.

Now, let's explore some delightful smoothie variations:

1. Berry Bliss: Blend a handful of mixed berries (strawberries, blueberries, raspberries) with Greek yogurt, a touch of honey, and a handful of spinach. This smoothie bursts with antioxidants and protein.

2. Tropical Paradise: Transport yourself to the tropics with a blend of mango, pineapple, coconut milk, and a scoop of vanilla protein powder. A pinch of turmeric adds a vibrant color and anti-inflammatory benefits.

3. Green Goddess: For a nutrient-packed green smoothie, combine spinach, kale, banana, avocado, and a spoonful of almond butter. This powerhouse smoothie is rich in vitamins, healthy fats, and fiber.

4. Peanut Butter Banana: A classic favorite, this smoothie pairs ripe bananas with peanut butter, Greek yogurt, and a dash of cinnamon. It's a creamy and protein-packed breakfast option.

5. Oatmeal Cookie: Capture the essence of a warm oatmeal cookie in a glass. Blend rolled oats, almond milk, a splash of vanilla extract, and a sprinkle of cinnamon. Add a banana or dates for natural sweetness.

6. Chocolate Delight: Satisfy your chocolate cravings with a cocoa-infused smoothie. Combine unsweetened cocoa powder, almond milk, a scoop of chocolate protein powder, and a handful of spinach for an extra nutritional boost.

7. Detoxifying Green Tea: Brew green tea and chill it overnight. In the morning, blend it with frozen pineapple, a handful of spinach, and a touch of honey for a refreshing and detoxifying start to your day.

Remember to experiment and adjust ingredient quantities to achieve your desired taste and consistency. Whether you're focused on weight management, increased energy, or simply enjoying a tasty breakfast, nutrient-packed smoothies offer endless possibilities for a healthy and satisfying morning meal. Start your day on a delicious and nutritious note with a custom-made breakfast smoothie!

Whole Grain Breakfast Ideas

Whole grains are a nutritional powerhouse, packed with fiber, vitamins, minerals, and complex carbohydrates that provide sustained energy throughout the morning. Incorporating whole grains into your breakfast not only keeps you full and satisfied but also contributes to your overall well-being. Let's explore a variety of delectable whole grain breakfast ideas that will elevate your morning routine.

1. Overnight Oats: Perhaps one of the most popular whole grain breakfast options, overnight oats are incredibly versatile and easy to prepare. Combine rolled oats with your choice of milk (dairy or non-dairy), sweetener, and toppings like fresh berries, nuts, and seeds. Let it sit in the fridge overnight, and in the morning, you have a creamy, nutritious breakfast ready to enjoy.

2. Quinoa Breakfast Bowls: Quinoa, a complete protein, makes an excellent base for breakfast bowls. Cook it in water or milk, add honey, cinnamon, and your favorite fruits (such as sliced banana, apple, or berries). Top it with a dollop of Greek yogurt for extra creaminess.

3. Whole Grain Pancakes: Swap out regular flour for whole wheat or oat flour when making pancakes. You can still enjoy fluffy pancakes but with the added benefit of whole grains. Top them with fresh fruit and a drizzle of pure maple syrup for a delicious morning treat.

4. Whole Grain Cereals: Opt for whole grain cereals like oatmeal, bran flakes, or whole wheat flakes. Enhance the flavor and nutrition by adding sliced almonds, chopped dates, and a dash of cinnamon. Remember to choose low-sugar or no-sugar-added options.

5. Homemade Granola: Create your own whole grain granola using rolled oats, nuts, seeds, and a touch of honey or maple syrup for sweetness. Bake until golden brown and crunchy. Serve it with yogurt and fresh fruit for a hearty breakfast.

6. Whole Grain Toast: Start your day with whole grain toast topped with avocado, a poached egg, and a sprinkle of crushed red pepper flakes. This combination offers a balance of healthy fats, protein, and whole grains.

7. Brown Rice Pudding: A twist on classic rice pudding, use brown rice instead of white for a nutritious breakfast. Cook the rice in milk, sweeten with a bit of honey or agave nectar, and add raisins and a pinch of cinnamon for flavor.

8. Chia Seed Pudding: Mix chia seeds with almond milk, a touch of vanilla extract, and a drizzle of honey. Let it sit overnight, and you'll wake up to a thick, pudding-like consistency that's perfect for layering with fruits, nuts, and granola.

9. Whole Grain Breakfast Burritos: Fill whole wheat tortillas with scrambled eggs, black beans, brown rice, and sautéed veggies. Roll them up and top with salsa for a savory and satisfying breakfast.

10. Farro Breakfast Bowl: Farro, a nutty and chewy whole grain, pairs wonderfully with roasted vegetables, poached eggs, and a drizzle of tahini or yogurt-based dressing.

Whole grains not only offer a spectrum of flavors but also diverse textures that can satisfy your morning cravings. Whether you're looking for a quick, on-the-go option or a leisurely weekend breakfast, these whole grain breakfast ideas will provide the nutrients and energy you need to start your day on the right foot. Incorporate them into your breakfast routine for a delicious and wholesome morning experience.

Creative Egg-Free Dishes

Eggs are a breakfast staple for many, but if you have allergies, dietary restrictions, or simply want to explore more diverse breakfast options, there's a world of egg-free breakfast dishes waiting to be discovered. These creative egg-free breakfast ideas are not only delicious but also packed with flavor and nutrients to kickstart your day with a smile.

1. Tofu Scramble: A vegan twist on scrambled eggs, tofu scramble is a protein-rich and satisfying alternative. Crumble firm tofu and sauté it with turmeric, nutritional yeast, vegetables, and your choice of spices for a savory breakfast dish that closely mimics the texture of scrambled eggs.

2. Chickpea Flour Pancakes: Chickpea flour, also known as besan or gram flour, is a versatile ingredient that can be used to make savory pancakes. Combine it with water, spices, and chopped veggies to create a savory pancake batter. Cook these pancakes until they're golden brown and enjoy a unique and satisfying breakfast.

3. Avocado Toast: Elevate the classic avocado toast by adding layers of flavor. Top your toast with mashed avocado, a sprinkle of red pepper flakes, a drizzle of olive oil, and a poached or fried tomato. The creamy avocado pairs perfectly with the tangy tomato.

4. Nut Butter and Banana Sandwich: Spread almond or peanut butter on whole grain bread and layer it with banana slices. You can add a drizzle of honey or a sprinkle of cinnamon for extra sweetness and flavor.

5. Breakfast Burritos with Tofu Scramble: Fill tortillas with tofu scramble, black beans, avocado, and salsa for a satisfying, protein-packed breakfast burrito that's completely egg-free.

6. Overnight Chia Pudding: Combine chia seeds with your choice of milk (almond, coconut, soy, etc.), a touch of vanilla extract, and a sweetener like honey or maple syrup. Let it sit in the fridge overnight, and you'll wake up to a thick, pudding-like breakfast. Top it with fresh fruit, nuts, and seeds.

7. Rice Cakes with Hummus and Veggies: Spread your favorite hummus on whole grain rice cakes and top them with sliced cucumbers, cherry tomatoes, and a sprinkle of everything bagel seasoning for a crunchy and savory breakfast.

8. Savory Oatmeal: Skip the sweet toppings and opt for savory oatmeal instead. Cook rolled oats with vegetable broth, sautéed spinach, mushrooms, and a sprinkle of nutritional yeast for a cheesy flavor.

9. Veggie Breakfast Wrap: Wrap sautéed spinach, roasted red pepper, and diced potatoes in a whole grain tortilla. Add a dollop of dairy-free yogurt or tahini sauce for extra creaminess.

10. Mediterranean Breakfast Plate: Create a Mediterranean-inspired breakfast by assembling a plate with olives, cucumber slices, cherry tomatoes, feta cheese (or dairy-free alternative), and a warm pita bread. Drizzle olive oil and sprinkle za'atar seasoning for an authentic touch.

These egg-free breakfast options offer variety, flavor, and nutrition, making your mornings more exciting and accommodating to your dietary preferences. Whether you're vegan, have egg allergies, or just want to try something new, these creative dishes will help you start your day with a delicious twist.

Chapter 4: Nourishing Lunches

Nourishing lunches are a vital component of a healthy and balanced diet. Whether you're a busy professional, a student, or someone who simply wants to maintain their well-being, taking the time to prepare and enjoy a nourishing lunch can make a significant difference in your overall health and productivity. In this article, we'll explore the importance of nourishing lunches, share some tips on how to create them, and provide a variety of delicious and nutritious lunch ideas to inspire your midday meals.

The Importance of Nourishing Lunches

A nourishing lunch serves as a midday energy boost, refueling your body and brain to power through the rest of the day. It should provide essential nutrients such as protein, fiber, vitamins, and minerals to support various bodily functions.

Here are some key benefits of incorporating nourishing lunches into your routine:

1. Sustained Energy: A well-balanced lunch can help maintain steady blood sugar levels, preventing energy crashes and that afternoon slump. It keeps you alert and focused.

2. Improved Concentration: Nutrient-rich lunches can enhance cognitive function, helping you think more clearly and make better decisions.

3. Weight Management: Eating a nourishing lunch can help control your appetite and reduce the likelihood of overindulging at dinner. It supports weight management and can aid in weight loss goals.

4. Digestive Health: A balanced lunch can promote healthy digestion and reduce the risk of digestive issues like bloating and discomfort.

5. Mood Regulation: Certain foods can influence mood and reduce the risk of mood swings or irritability. A nourishing lunch can contribute to a positive mental state.

Tips for Creating Nourishing Lunches

Creating nourishing lunches doesn't have to be complicated or time-consuming. Here are some tips to help you build a satisfying and nutritious midday meal:

1. Balance Macronutrients: Include a source of lean protein (e.g., chicken, tofu, beans), complex carbohydrates (e.g., whole grains, sweet potatoes), and healthy fats (e.g., avocado, nuts) in your lunch to ensure a balanced meal.

2. Load Up on Veggies: Vegetables are packed with vitamins, minerals, and fiber. Incorporate a variety of colorful vegetables to maximize nutrition.

3. Minimize Processed Foods: Limit processed and sugary foods, such as chips and soda. Opt for whole, unprocessed ingredients whenever possible.

4. Portion Control: Be mindful of portion sizes to avoid overeating. Use smaller plates or containers to help with portion control.

5. Stay Hydrated: Don't forget to drink water throughout the day. Dehydration can sometimes be mistaken for hunger.

6. Meal Prep: Plan and prepare your lunches in advance to save time during busy weekdays. Having healthy options readily available can prevent you from reaching for unhealthy alternatives.

Nourishing Lunch Ideas

Now that we've covered the importance of nourishing lunches and how to create them, here are some delicious and nutritious lunch ideas to inspire your midday meals:

1. Grilled Chicken and Quinoa Salad: A colorful salad with grilled chicken, quinoa, cherry tomatoes, cucumbers, and a lemon vinaigrette.

2. Vegetable Stir-Fry: Stir-fry a mix of colorful vegetables with tofu or lean protein and serve over brown rice or cauliflower rice.

3. Sweet Potato and Black Bean Bowl: Roasted sweet potatoes, black beans, avocado, and salsa make a hearty and flavorful lunch.

4. Greek Yogurt Parfait: Layer Greek yogurt with granola, berries, and honey for a protein-packed and satisfying lunch.

5. Salmon and Asparagus: Baked salmon with roasted asparagus and a side of quinoa is a quick and nutritious option.

6. Mediterranean Wrap: Fill a whole-grain wrap with hummus, roasted vegetables, olives, and feta cheese.

7. Minestrone Soup: A hearty vegetable and bean soup is perfect for a comforting and nourishing lunch.

The key to a nourishing lunch is variety and balance. Experiment with different ingredients, flavors, and cuisines to keep your lunches exciting and packed with nutrients. By prioritizing nourishing lunches, you'll be taking a proactive step toward better health and well-being.

Wholesome Salads

Salads are often associated with light and refreshing meals, but they can be incredibly nourishing and satisfying when prepared thoughtfully. Wholesome salads can provide a delightful array of flavors, textures, and nutrients in a single bowl, making them an excellent choice for a nourishing lunch. In this article, we will explore the art of creating wholesome salads that not only taste delicious but also provide your body with essential nutrients.

The Foundation of Wholesome Salads

A truly nourishing salad begins with a solid foundation of fresh, nutrient-rich greens. While iceberg lettuce may be the first thing that comes to mind, consider branching out to more nutrient-dense options like:

1. Spinach: Packed with iron, fiber, and vitamins A and K, spinach is a nutritious base for any salad.

2. Kale: Known for its exceptional vitamin content, particularly vitamin K and vitamin C, kale adds a hearty, earthy flavor.

3. Arugula: Offering a peppery kick, arugula is a great source of antioxidants and vitamins.

4. Romaine Lettuce: Crisp and refreshing, romaine lettuce is a low-calorie option with vitamins A and K.

5. Mixed Greens: A mix of various greens, like mesclun or spring mix, provides a medley of flavors and nutrients.

The Art of Toppings

Toppings are where the magic happens in a salad. They add flavor, texture, and a diverse range of nutrients. Here are some nourishing topping options to consider:

1. Proteins: Add lean proteins like grilled chicken, tofu, chickpeas, or quinoa for satiety and muscle repair.

2. Healthy Fats: Avocado slices, nuts (such as almonds or walnuts), and seeds (like chia or flaxseed) provide heart-healthy fats.

3. Colorful Vegetables: Load up your salad with a rainbow of vegetables like bell peppers, cherry tomatoes, cucumbers, carrots, and red onions for vitamins, minerals, and antioxidants.

4. Fruits: Fresh or dried fruits like berries, apples, or raisins add natural sweetness and extra fiber.

5. Cheeses: Opt for small amounts of flavorful, lower-fat cheeses like feta, goat cheese, or Parmesan for richness.

6. Herbs and Fresh Herbs: Add fresh herbs like basil, cilantro, or mint for an aromatic burst of flavor.

Dressing it Up

The dressing can make or break your salad, so choose wisely. Homemade dressings are often healthier and tastier than store-bought ones, as they allow you to control the ingredients. Some nourishing dressing options include:

1. Olive Oil and Balsamic Vinegar: A classic and simple combination that provides healthy fats and tangy flavor.

2. Greek Yogurt: Use yogurt as a base for a creamy dressing that's lower in calories but still rich in flavor.

3. Lemon or Lime Vinaigrette: Fresh citrus juice mixed with olive oil, Dijon mustard, and herbs creates a zesty and light dressing.

4. Tahini: This sesame paste-based dressing offers a unique nutty flavor and creaminess.

5. Honey Mustard: Combine Dijon mustard, honey, and a touch of vinegar for a sweet and tangy dressing.

Building a Balanced Salad

To ensure that your salad is truly nourishing and balanced, aim to include a variety of elements:

- **Protein:** A good source of lean protein, whether it's plant-based or animal protein, to keep you full and satisfied.

- **Fiber:** Load up on fiber-rich vegetables, fruits, and whole grains to aid digestion and provide long-lasting energy.

- Healthy Fats: Incorporate sources of healthy fats like avocado, nuts, seeds, or olive oil for satiety and overall well-being.

- Color Variety: Aim for a colorful mix of ingredients to ensure a wide range of vitamins, minerals, and antioxidants.

By mastering the art of crafting nourishing salads, you can transform a seemingly simple meal into a wholesome, nutrient-packed lunch that leaves you feeling satisfied and energized throughout the day. Experiment with different ingredients, textures, and flavors to discover your favorite combinations, and enjoy the benefits of nourishing salads as a regular part of your lunchtime routine.

Hearty Soups

Hearty soups are a comforting and nourishing lunch option that can warm your body and soul, especially on chilly days. These savory concoctions offer a wealth of flavors and textures while providing essential nutrients to keep you satisfied and energized. In this article, we'll explore the world of hearty soups, discuss their benefits, and share some delicious recipes to inspire your lunchtime choices.

The Appeal of Hearty Soups

Hearty soups are more than just a bowl of warm liquid; they are a wholesome meal in themselves. Here are some reasons why hearty soups make an excellent choice for nourishing lunches:

1. **Nutrient Density:** Soups often contain a variety of vegetables, proteins, and grains, making them nutrient-dense. They provide essential vitamins, minerals, and fiber in a single bowl.

2. **Satiety:** The combination of liquid and solid components in soups can help you feel full and satisfied, reducing the likelihood of overeating later in the day.

3. Hydration: Soups contain water, which contributes to your daily hydration needs, ensuring you stay well-hydrated.

4. Easy Digestion: The cooking process breaks down ingredients, making nutrients more accessible and easier to digest, which can be especially beneficial for individuals with digestive sensitivities.

5. Endless Varieties: Soups can be customized to suit your taste preferences and dietary requirements, allowing for endless flavor combinations.

Tips for Creating Hearty Soups

Creating a hearty and nourishing soup doesn't require advanced culinary skills. Here are some tips to help you craft a satisfying bowl of soup:

1. Start with a Flavorful Base: Begin by sautéing aromatics like onions, garlic, and spices to build a flavorful base for your soup.

2. Balance Ingredients: Include a mix of vegetables, proteins (such as beans, chicken, or tofu), and grains (like pasta, rice, or barley) to create a well-balanced soup.

3. Homemade Broth: Whenever possible, opt for homemade broth or stock, as it allows you to control the sodium content and flavor profile.

4. Fresh Herbs and Seasoning: Fresh herbs like basil, thyme, or cilantro, and seasonings like salt and pepper, can elevate the taste of your soup.

5. Texture Variation: Add ingredients at different times to vary the soup's texture. For example, add vegetables at the beginning and fresh herbs at the end.

6. Healthy Fats: Incorporate healthy fats like olive oil or avocado to enhance the richness and mouthfeel of your soup.

Hearty Soup Recipes

Now, let's explore some hearty soup recipes that are both nourishing and delicious:

1. Chicken and Vegetable Soup: Simmer chicken breast, carrots, celery, onions, and whole wheat noodles in chicken broth for a classic, comforting soup.

2. Vegetarian Minestrone: A medley of vegetables, kidney beans, pasta, and herbs in a tomato-based broth creates a hearty and nutritious soup.

3. Lentil and Kale Soup: Red lentils, kale, tomatoes, and spices combine to form a protein-packed, plant-based soup.

4. Creamy Butternut Squash Soup: Roasted butternut squash blended with coconut milk and warming spices results in a creamy and comforting soup.

5. Tom Kha Gai (Thai Coconut Soup): This aromatic soup features coconut milk, chicken, mushrooms, and lemongrass for a delightful fusion of flavors.

6. Black Bean Chili: A hearty and spicy chili loaded with black beans, vegetables, and a variety of spices makes for a filling and nourishing meal.

The beauty of hearty soups lies in their adaptability. Feel free to experiment with ingredients, adjust flavors to your liking, and tailor the soups to your dietary preferences. Whether you're a fan of classic chicken soup or prefer vegan options, hearty soups offer a satisfying and nutritious lunch option that can easily become a staple in your meal rotation.

Chapter 5: Satisfying Dinners

Dinner is more than just a meal; it's a moment of satisfaction, a time to unwind, and an opportunity to nourish both body and soul. Whether you're preparing a weeknight dinner for your family or hosting a special gathering with friends, the quest for a satisfying dinner is universal. In this culinary journey, we'll explore the art of creating dinners that not only fill your belly but also leave you with a sense of contentment and delight.

The Essentials of a Satisfying Dinner:

1. Balanced Nutrition: A satisfying dinner starts with a well-rounded plate. Incorporate a variety of food groups, including lean proteins, colorful vegetables, whole grains, and healthy fats. This balance ensures you're not only satisfying your taste buds but also meeting your nutritional needs.

2. Flavor Harmony: The key to a memorable dinner lies in achieving the right balance of flavors. Sweet, salty, sour, bitter, and umami - these tastes should harmonize in your dish. Experiment with herbs, spices, and condiments to elevate the flavors to a whole new level.

3. Texture Play: Texture can transform a mundane meal into a satisfying experience. Think about the contrast between crispy, crunchy, and tender. Pair crispy roasted vegetables with a succulent, slow-cooked protein, or add a sprinkle of toasted nuts for an extra layer of satisfaction.

4. Presentation Matters: They say we eat with our eyes first, and it's true. A beautifully plated dinner not only looks enticing but also enhances the dining experience. Take time to garnish and arrange your dish thoughtfully.

Satisfying Dinner Ideas:

1. Classic Comfort Food: Sometimes, a hearty plate of comfort food is all you need to satisfy your cravings. Think mac and cheese, a rich lasagna, or a bowl of creamy tomato soup paired with a grilled cheese sandwich.

2. International Delights: Explore the world through your dinner plate. Try your hand at making authentic Italian pasta dishes, flavorful Thai curries, or mouthwatering Indian cuisine. The flavors of global cuisines can transport you to distant lands, leaving you utterly satisfied.

3. Grilled Goodness: Firing up the grill adds a smoky depth to your dinner. Grilled chicken, steak, or even vegetables with a touch of char bring a unique satisfaction that's hard to beat.

4. One-Pot Wonders: Simplify your dinner routine with one-pot meals. Whether it's a hearty chili, a fragrant risotto, or a savory stir-fry, these dishes not only satisfy your hunger but also save you from a mountain of dishes.

5. Vegetarian and Vegan Delights: Satisfying dinners need not always revolve around meat.

Explore the world of plant-based cuisine with dishes like stuffed bell peppers, lentil shepherd's pie, or a comforting bowl of vegetable curry.

6. Seafood Sensations: Fresh seafood can be the star of your dinner table. Grilled salmon with a lemon dill sauce, shrimp scampi, or a seafood paella can bring coastal satisfaction to your home.

7. Homemade Pizza: There's something undeniably satisfying about crafting your pizza from scratch. Experiment with toppings, sauces, and crusts to create your ultimate pizza masterpiece.

The most satisfying dinners are those shared with loved ones. The joy of cooking and eating together adds an extra layer of fulfillment to the meal. So, whether you're planning a romantic dinner for two or a feast for a crowd, put thought and care into your dinner preparation. Embrace the process, savor the flavors, and relish the satisfaction that a well-prepared dinner can bring to your life.

Plant-Based Protein Recipes

In recent years, the popularity of plant-based diets has soared, and for a good reason. Not only are these diets environmentally friendly, but they also offer numerous health benefits. One common misconception, however, is that plant-based dinners lack protein and are unsatisfying. This couldn't be further from the truth. With the right ingredients and recipes, plant-based dinners can be not only nutritious but also incredibly satisfying. Let's explore some mouthwatering plant-based protein recipes that will leave you feeling full and content.

1. Chickpea and Spinach Curry:

This hearty and flavorful dish is packed with plant-based protein and essential nutrients.

Ingredients:

- 1 can of chickpeas, drained and rinsed

- 2 cups of fresh spinach

- 1 onion, finely chopped

- 3 cloves of garlic, minced

- 1 can of diced tomatoes

- 1 can of coconut milk

- 2 tablespoons of curry powder

- Salt and pepper to taste

- Olive oil for cooking

Instructions:

1. Heat olive oil in a large pan, and sauté the chopped onions and garlic until translucent.

2. Add the curry powder and cook for another minute to release its aroma.

3. Pour in the diced tomatoes, coconut milk, and chickpeas. Stir well and let it simmer for about 15 minutes, allowing the flavors to meld.

4. Add the fresh spinach and cook until wilted.

5. Season with salt and pepper to taste. Serve over brown rice or with naan bread for a satisfying dinner.

2. Lentil and Mushroom Stuffed Bell Peppers:

These stuffed bell peppers are not only visually appealing but also protein-packed and delicious.

Ingredients:

- 4 large bell peppers, any color
- 1 cup of brown or green lentils, cooked
- 1 cup of mushrooms, finely chopped
- 1 small onion, diced
- 2 cloves of garlic, minced
- 1 can of tomato sauce
- 1 teaspoon of Italian seasoning
- Salt and pepper to taste
- Olive oil for cooking

Instructions:

1. Preheat your oven to 375°F (190°C).

2. Cut the tops off the bell peppers and remove the seeds and membranes. Set aside.

3. In a large skillet, heat olive oil over medium heat. Add the chopped onions, garlic, and mushrooms, and sauté until softened.

4. Stir in the cooked lentils, Italian seasoning, and half of the tomato sauce. Season with salt and pepper.

5. Fill the bell peppers with the lentil-mushroom mixture and place them in a baking dish.

6. Pour the remaining tomato sauce over the stuffed peppers.

7. Cover the dish with aluminum foil and bake for 25-30 minutes, or until the peppers are tender.

8. Serve hot, and enjoy your protein-packed plant-based dinner!

3. Tofu and Vegetable Stir-Fry:

Stir-fries are quick, versatile, and perfect for adding plant-based protein.

Ingredients:

- 1 block of firm tofu, cubed
- 2 cups of mixed vegetables (bell peppers, broccoli, snap peas, carrots, etc.), sliced
- 2 cloves of garlic, minced
- 1 tablespoon of ginger, minced
- 3 tablespoons of soy sauce
- 1 tablespoon of sesame oil
- 1 tablespoon of cornstarch
- Cooked rice or noodles for serving

Instructions:

1. In a small bowl, whisk together the soy sauce, sesame oil, and cornstarch to make the sauce. Set aside.

2. Heat a large skillet or wok over medium-high heat and add a bit of oil.

3. Add the cubed tofu and stir-fry until it's lightly browned on all sides. Remove the tofu from the skillet and set it aside.

4. In the same skillet, add a bit more oil if needed, and stir-fry the minced garlic and ginger for about 30 seconds.

5. Add the sliced vegetables and continue to stir-fry until they're tender-crisp.

6. Return the tofu to the skillet and pour the sauce over everything. Stir-fry for another couple of minutes until the sauce thickens.

7. Serve your tofu and vegetable stir-fry over cooked rice or noodles for a satisfying and protein-rich dinner.

These plant-based protein recipes prove that you don't need meat to create delicious and fulfilling dinners. Whether you're a dedicated vegan or simply looking to incorporate more plant-based meals into your diet, these recipes will leave your taste buds delighted and your body nourished. Enjoy the journey of exploring new flavors and the satisfaction of knowing you're making a positive impact on your health and the planet.

Flavorful Vegetable-Centric Dishes

Vegetable-centric dinners have taken center stage in recent years as more people seek to incorporate the bounty of fresh produce into their daily meals. These dishes not only celebrate the vibrant colors and textures of vegetables but also deliver a burst of flavor that satisfies the palate. Whether you're a dedicated vegetarian, looking to reduce your meat consumption, or simply craving a hearty vegetable-focused meal, these flavorful recipes will leave you feeling fulfilled and nourished.

1. Roasted Vegetable Medley:

A simple yet incredibly satisfying dish, roasted vegetable medleys allow the natural flavors of vegetables to shine.

Ingredients:

- An assortment of your favorite vegetables (e.g., carrots, bell peppers, zucchini, cherry tomatoes, broccoli, and red onion)
- Olive oil
- Fresh herbs (rosemary, thyme, or basil)
- Salt and pepper to taste

Instructions:

1. Preheat your oven to 400°F (200°C).

2. Wash, peel (if necessary), and chop the vegetables into bite-sized pieces.

3. Toss the vegetables in olive oil, fresh herbs, salt, and pepper.

4. Spread them evenly on a baking sheet and roast for about 20-25 minutes or until they are tender and slightly caramelized.

5. Serve as a side dish or over cooked quinoa or couscous for a complete and satisfying dinner.

2. Stuffed Bell Peppers:

Stuffed bell peppers are a classic vegetable-centric dinner that combines nutrition and flavor.

Ingredients:

- Bell peppers (any color)
- Cooked quinoa or rice
- A mix of sautéed vegetables (e.g., mushrooms, spinach, tomatoes, and onions)
- Your choice of protein (tofu, beans, or lentils)
- Spices and seasonings of your choice
- Tomato sauce or marinara for topping

Instructions:

1. Cut the tops off the bell peppers and remove the seeds and membranes.

2. In a bowl, combine cooked quinoa or rice, sautéed vegetables, your choice of protein, and your favorite seasonings.

3. Stuff the bell peppers with this mixture.

4. Place the stuffed peppers in a baking dish, pour tomato sauce or marinara over them, and bake at 350°F (175°C) for 30-35 minutes, or until the peppers are tender.

5. Enjoy your wholesome and flavorful stuffed bell peppers!

3. Creamy Butternut Squash Soup:

A creamy butternut squash soup is the epitome of comfort and satisfaction on a chilly evening.

Ingredients:

- 1 medium butternut squash, peeled, seeded, and diced
- 1 onion, chopped
- 2 cloves of garlic, minced
- Vegetable broth
- Coconut milk or cream
- Ground nutmeg, cinnamon, salt, and pepper to taste

Instructions:

1. In a large pot, sauté the chopped onion and garlic until they're soft and translucent.

2. Add the diced butternut squash and continue to sauté for a few more minutes.

3. Pour in enough vegetable broth to cover the squash, and bring it to a boil. Reduce the heat and simmer until the squash is tender.

4. Use an immersion blender or a regular blender to puree the soup until smooth.

5. Stir in a bit of coconut milk or cream for creaminess, and season with ground nutmeg, cinnamon, salt, and pepper.

6. Serve hot, and garnish with a drizzle of coconut milk and a sprinkle of fresh herbs or roasted pumpkin seeds.

These vegetable-centric dishes prove that plant-based dinners can be both satisfying and bursting with flavor. Whether you're embracing a vegetarian lifestyle or simply looking to add more vegetables to your diet, these recipes will not only tantalize your taste buds but also leave you feeling nourished and content. Celebrate the delicious world of vegetables and enjoy the satisfaction of savoring their natural goodness.

Dinner Prep and Cooking Tips

Preparing and cooking a satisfying dinner can be a joyful experience, but it can also be a bit challenging, especially if you're pressed for time or unsure of your culinary skills. However, with some planning, organization, and a few cooking tips, you can create delicious and satisfying dinners that leave you and your loved ones wanting more. Here are some valuable dinner prep and cooking tips to make your evening meals a breeze.

1. Plan Your Meals in Advance:

- Start your dinner journey with a well-thought-out meal plan for the week. This can help you ensure balanced nutrition, reduce food waste, and make grocery shopping a breeze.

2. Stock Your Kitchen:

- Keep your pantry and refrigerator well-stocked with essential ingredients like olive oil, various spices, canned tomatoes, pasta, rice, beans, and a variety of fresh vegetables and proteins. Having these staples on hand makes it easier to whip up satisfying dinners on short notice.

3. Prep Ahead of Time:

- Spend some time on meal prep during the weekend or whenever you have some free time. Chop vegetables, marinate proteins, or make sauces in advance. This can save you precious minutes on busy weeknights.

4. Invest in Quality Cookware:

- Having the right cookware can make a significant difference in your cooking experience. Invest in good-quality pots, pans, knives, and utensils to make dinner preparation more efficient and enjoyable.

5. Timing Is Key:

- Plan your cooking time wisely. Start with tasks that require the most time, like preheating the oven or simmering a stew, and then work on other components of the meal while these are cooking.

6. Don't Neglect Seasonings:

- Season your dishes throughout the cooking process, not just at the end. This allows the flavors to meld together and ensures your dinner is well-seasoned and satisfying.

7. Master the Art of Searing:

- Achieving a good sear on proteins and vegetables adds depth and flavor to your dishes. Make sure your pan is hot and dry before adding ingredients to get that satisfying caramelization.

8. Embrace One-Pot and Sheet Pan Meals:

- One-pot and sheet pan dinners can be lifesavers on busy evenings. They reduce cleanup time and often yield delicious, well-balanced meals.

9. Taste as You Go:

- Regularly taste your food as you cook. Adjust seasonings, add more spices, or make flavor enhancements as needed to ensure the final dish is satisfying.

10. Use Fresh Herbs and Citrus:

- Fresh herbs like basil, cilantro, and parsley, along with a squeeze of citrus (lemon, lime, or orange), can elevate the flavors of your dinner and add a refreshing touch.

11. Learn Basic Cooking Techniques:

- Mastering basic cooking techniques like sautéing, braising, roasting, and grilling can open up a world of possibilities for creating satisfying dinners.

12. Balance Your Plate:

- Aim for a balanced plate that includes protein, vegetables, and a carbohydrate source like grains or legumes. This ensures your dinner is both satisfying and nutritious.

13. Don't Forget About Presentation:

- A beautifully plated dinner not only looks more appealing but also enhances your dining experience. Take a moment to arrange your food thoughtfully on the plate.

14. Experiment and Have Fun:

- Don't be afraid to get creative in the kitchen. Experiment with new ingredients, flavors, and cuisines to keep dinner exciting and satisfying.

cooking is a skill that improves with practice, so don't be discouraged if your first attempts aren't perfect. The key is to enjoy the process and savor the satisfaction that comes from creating and sharing a delicious dinner. Happy cooking!

Chapter 6: Snacks, Sides, and Desserts

In the world of gastronomy, there's a delightful trio that often steals the show, offering an array of flavors and textures that can satisfy every craving. Snacks, sides, and desserts, while distinct in their roles, collectively contribute to the overall dining experience, turning an ordinary meal into a memorable feast. Let's explore each of these culinary categories and discover the magic they bring to our tables.

1. Snacks: Small Bites with Big Impact

Snacks are the unsung heroes of the culinary world. These small bites hold the power to satiate your hunger between meals, add a burst of flavor to gatherings, or simply provide a moment of indulgence during a hectic day. From crispy potato chips to savory samosas, snacks come in various forms and flavors, making them a diverse category in the culinary realm.

a. Savory Snacks:

- **Chips and Crisps:** Whether it's classic potato chips, tortilla chips, or gourmet vegetable crisps, the satisfying crunch and salty goodness of these snacks are hard to resist.

- **Dips and Salsas:** Pair your chips with creamy guacamole, spicy salsa, or a tangy tzatziki for an explosion of flavors.

- **Fried Delights:** Think of samosas, spring rolls, or tempura as crispy parcels filled with a variety of ingredients, from vegetables to meats.

b. Sweet Snacks:

- **Candies and Chocolates:** From gummy bears to artisanal chocolates, sweet snacks offer a sugar rush that can brighten up your day.

- **Cookies and Biscuits:** These baked delights come in countless flavors and textures, from soft and chewy to crispy and buttery.

- **Fruit Snacks:** Nature's candy, dried fruits, fruit leather, and fruit gummies provide a healthy and sweet alternative.

2. Sides: The Perfect Companions

Sides, also known as side dishes, are the supporting actors in a meal, enhancing the main course's flavors and providing balance. They can be the difference between a mundane dinner and a memorable one, transforming a simple plate of food into a well-rounded culinary experience.

a. Vegetables: Sides like roasted vegetables, buttery mashed potatoes, or sautéed greens add color, nutrition, and a range of tastes and textures to your plate.

b. Grains: Rice, quinoa, couscous, and pasta make for versatile sides that can complement a variety of dishes.

c. Breads: Freshly baked bread, rolls, or naan can be the perfect accompaniment to soups, stews, or curries.

d. Sauces and Condiments: From tangy barbecue sauces to creamy aioli, these add layers of flavor and complexity to your meal.

3. Desserts: Sweet Endings

Desserts are the grand finale of any meal, designed to indulge your sweet tooth and leave a lasting impression. Whether it's a decadent chocolate cake, a fruity tart, or a scoop of ice cream, desserts are the crowning glory of culinary creativity.

a. Cakes and Pastries: Layered cakes, cheesecakes, éclairs, and tarts showcase the artistry of pastry chefs and bakers.

b. Pies and Cobblers: Fruit-filled pies, cobblers, and crisps evoke a comforting, homey feeling with each bite.

c. Frozen Treats: Ice cream, gelato, and sorbet offer a refreshing, cool sweetness, making them a favorite during hot summer months.

d. Custards and Puddings: Creamy and comforting, custards, flans, and puddings are timeless classics that delight with every spoonful.

Snacks, sides, and desserts play crucial roles in the world of cuisine, each offering a unique set of flavors, textures, and experiences. Whether you're enjoying a quick snack on the go, savoring the perfect side dish, or indulging in a decadent dessert, these culinary delights enrich our lives, making every meal a celebration of taste and pleasure. So, next time you sit down to dine, remember to embrace the magic of snacks, sides, and desserts that transform an ordinary meal into an extraordinary one.

Healthy Snacking Choices

In a world where convenience often leads to unhealthy eating habits, making smart choices when it comes to snacks is more important than ever. Snacking doesn't have to be synonymous with guilt and regret. With the right approach, you can enjoy delicious and satisfying snacks that not only curb your cravings but also contribute to your overall well-being. Let's explore some healthy snacking choices within the realm of snacks, sides, and desserts.

1. Snacks: Nourishing Bites

When it comes to snacks, opting for nutritious options can be a game-changer for your health. These snacks provide a boost of energy, essential nutrients, and can even help you stay fuller for longer.

a. Fresh Fruits and Vegetables:

- **Sliced Apples with Peanut Butter:** The combination of fiber-rich apples and protein-packed peanut butter is both satisfying and nutritious.

- **Carrot and Cucumber Sticks with Hummus:** Crunchy veggies paired with creamy hummus make for a refreshing and low-calorie snack.

- **Berries and Greek Yogurt:** A bowl of fresh berries with a dollop of Greek yogurt offers antioxidants and protein.

b. Nuts and Seeds:

- **Almonds, Walnuts, and Cashews:** These nuts are packed with healthy fats, fiber, and protein. A small handful can keep you satisfied.

- **Chia Pudding:** Mix chia seeds with almond milk and a touch of honey for a nutritious, fiber-rich pudding.

c. Whole Grains:

- **Popcorn:** Air-popped popcorn is a whole-grain snack that's low in calories and high in fiber.

- **Whole Grain Crackers with Avocado:** Top whole-grain crackers with slices of avocado for a creamy, satisfying snack.

2. Sides: Balancing Your Plate

Sides can be more than just add-ons to your meal; they can be nutrient-rich components that enhance your overall dietary intake.

a. Roasted Vegetables:

- **Roasted Brussels Sprouts:** Seasoned with olive oil and herbs, these are not only delicious but also rich in vitamins and fiber.

- **Sweet Potato Fries:** Satisfy your cravings for something crispy with sweet potato fries, a healthier alternative to regular fries.

b. Grains:

- **Quinoa Salad:** A cold quinoa salad with veggies and a light vinaigrette is a nutritious side that's also filling.

- **Brown Rice with Stir-Fried Tofu:** High in protein and fiber, this combination is both wholesome and satisfying.

c. Legumes:

- **Hummus and Veggie Platter:** A colorful array of sliced vegetables with hummus is a fiber and protein-packed side.

- **Black Bean Salad:** A zesty black bean salad with corn, peppers, and lime dressing is a delicious and nutritious option.

3. Desserts: Sweet Indulgences with a Healthy Twist

Desserts can be enjoyed without derailing your healthy eating goals. There are numerous ways to create sweet treats that satisfy your cravings while staying mindful of your well-being.

a. Fruit-Based Desserts:

- **Fruit Salad:** A medley of fresh, ripe fruits drizzled with a touch of honey or a sprinkle of cinnamon can be a delightful dessert.

- **Baked Apples:** Baking apples with a dash of cinnamon and a drizzle of maple syrup results in a warm, naturally sweet treat.

b. Yogurt Parfaits:

- **Greek Yogurt Parfait:** Layer Greek yogurt with berries, nuts, and a drizzle of honey for a protein-packed dessert.

- **Chia Seed Pudding:** Combine chia seeds, almond milk, and your favorite fruit for a creamy, nutritious pudding.

c. Dark Chocolate:

   - **Dark Chocolate Covered Almonds:** Dark chocolate with almonds offers antioxidants and satisfies chocolate cravings in moderation.

   - **Chocolate-Dipped Strawberries:** A few chocolate-dipped strawberries can provide a sweet ending to your meal.

Incorporating these healthy snacking choices into your daily routine can help you maintain a balanced diet while still enjoying the pleasures of snacks, sides, and desserts. Remember, it's all about making mindful choices and finding delicious alternatives that nourish your body and soul.

Appetizing Side Dishes

Side dishes play a pivotal role in elevating a meal from ordinary to extraordinary. These culinary accompaniments not only provide balance and contrast to the main course but also introduce an exciting array of flavors, textures, and colors to the dining experience. Whether you're hosting a dinner party or simply preparing a family meal, crafting appetizing side dishes can take your culinary prowess to the next level.

Let's delve into the world of appetizing side dishes, exploring various options to complement different cuisines and occasions.

1. Vegetable Side Dishes: A Symphony of Flavors

Vegetables are often the stars of side dishes, offering an opportunity to showcase their natural flavors and textures. Here are some delectable options:

a. Roasted Vegetables: Oven-roasting brings out the natural sweetness and caramelization of vegetables like carrots, Brussels sprouts, and butternut squash. A drizzle of olive oil and a sprinkle of herbs can make them irresistible.

b. Garlic and Herb Mashed Potatoes: Creamy mashed potatoes infused with roasted garlic and fresh herbs provide a comforting and flavorful side for various main courses.

c. Sautéed Greens: Spinach, kale, or Swiss chard sautéed with garlic and olive oil is a nutritious and vibrant side dish that pairs well with grilled proteins.

d. Ratatouille: This classic French dish combines a medley of eggplant, zucchini, bell peppers, and tomatoes, simmered with aromatic herbs and garlic for a colorful and flavorful side.

2. Grain-Based Side Dishes: Wholesome and Satisfying

Grains are versatile and can serve as the foundation for appetizing side dishes. They provide substance and can be adapted to complement different cuisines:

a. Fried Rice: A fragrant mix of cooked rice, vegetables, and proteins (such as shrimp or tofu) stir-fried with soy sauce and seasonings creates a satisfying side dish or even a standalone meal.

b. Couscous Salad: Light and fluffy couscous tossed with colorful bell peppers, cherry tomatoes, cucumber, and fresh herbs, dressed with lemon vinaigrette, is a refreshing and Mediterranean-inspired side.

c. Quinoa Pilaf: Nutty quinoa cooked with sautéed onions, toasted almonds, and dried fruits like cranberries or apricots makes for an enticing and wholesome side.

d. Polenta: Creamy polenta topped with sautéed mushrooms, a rich tomato sauce, or a sprinkle of Parmesan cheese is a comforting and hearty accompaniment.

3. Bread and Pastry Sides: Comforting Classics

Breads and pastries offer a delightful addition to any meal, often bringing warmth and comfort to the table:

a. Garlic Bread: Slices of crusty bread slathered with garlic butter and baked until golden brown are the perfect side for pasta dishes and Italian cuisine.

b. Cornbread: This sweet and savory bread pairs wonderfully with chili, barbecue, or Southern-style meals, and it's easily customizable with ingredients like jalapeños or cheese.

c. Puff Pastry Tarts: Puff pastry sheets filled with ingredients like caramelized onions, goat cheese, and roasted vegetables can be cut into elegant squares or slices for an impressive side.

4. Salad Sides: Fresh and Vibrant Choices

Salads are versatile and can be adapted to match the flavors of your main course. They provide a refreshing contrast to heartier dishes:

a. Caprese Salad: Slices of ripe tomatoes, fresh mozzarella cheese, basil leaves, and a drizzle of balsamic glaze create a classic Italian side that celebrates simplicity and quality ingredients.

b. **Caesar Salad:** Crisp romaine lettuce, homemade croutons, Parmesan cheese, and a creamy Caesar dressing result in a timeless and flavorful accompaniment.

c. Asian Slaw: A crunchy and colorful coleslaw with a sesame ginger dressing pairs beautifully with Asian-inspired dishes, grilled meats, or seafood.

d. Fruit Salad: A medley of fresh fruits like melons, berries, and citrus segments offers a sweet and refreshing side for brunches or warm-weather gatherings.

Appetizing side dishes have the power to elevate your dining experience, adding depth and dimension to your meals. Whether you're aiming for comfort, sophistication, or a burst of freshness, the world of side dishes offers endless possibilities to tantalize your taste buds and impress your guests. So, the next time you prepare a meal, don't underestimate the impact of a well-crafted side dish—it might just steal the show!

Guilt-Free Dessert Options

Desserts are often considered a guilty pleasure, and for a good reason. Traditional desserts are laden with sugar, fats, and empty calories that can derail even the healthiest of diets. However, indulging in a sweet treat doesn't have to come at the cost of your health and well-being. There are plenty of guilt-free dessert options that allow you to satisfy your sweet tooth while still nourishing your body. Let's explore some of these delicious and wholesome alternatives:

1. Fruit-Centric Desserts: Nature's Candy

Fruits are a natural source of sweetness, and they provide essential vitamins, fiber, and antioxidants. Harness the power of nature's candy with these guilt-free dessert ideas:

a. Fruit Salad: A colorful medley of fresh fruits like berries, melons, and citrus segments drizzled with a touch of honey or a sprinkle of cinnamon can be a delightful and nutritious dessert.

b. Baked Apples: Core and stuff apples with a mixture of oats, cinnamon, and a drizzle of maple syrup, then bake until tender for a warm, naturally sweet treat.

c. Frozen Banana "Ice Cream": Freeze ripe bananas, then blend them until creamy. Add a dash of vanilla extract or cocoa powder for flavor variations. It's a dairy-free and sugar-free alternative to traditional ice cream.

2. Yogurt-Based Treats: Creamy and Wholesome

Yogurt is a versatile ingredient that can be transformed into various guilt-free dessert options:

a. Greek Yogurt Parfait: Layer Greek yogurt with fresh berries, nuts, and a drizzle of honey for a protein-packed and satisfying dessert.

b. Yogurt Popsicles: Mix yogurt with pureed fruit, pour the mixture into popsicle molds, and freeze. These homemade popsicles are a refreshing and low-calorie summer treat.

c. Yogurt and Honey Dip: Create a creamy dip by mixing Greek yogurt with honey and a pinch of cinnamon. Serve with slices of apple or pear for a delightful, guilt-free snack.

3. Dark Chocolate Delights: The Bittersweet Solution

Dark chocolate, with a high cocoa content, offers the richness of chocolate without the excessive sugar and unhealthy fats:

a. Dark Chocolate-Covered Almonds: A small handful of almonds coated in dark chocolate not only satisfies your sweet cravings but also provides a dose of healthy fats and antioxidants.

b. Chocolate-Dipped Strawberries: A classic favorite, strawberries dipped in dark chocolate are an elegant and guilt-free dessert option.

4. Nut and Seed-Based Desserts: Healthy Crunch

Nuts and seeds are packed with nutrients, healthy fats, and proteins, making them ideal candidates for guilt-free desserts:

a. Energy Bites: Combine nuts, seeds, dried fruits, and a touch of honey or nut butter to create bite-sized energy balls that are perfect for on-the-go snacking or dessert.

b. Almond Butter Cups: Swap traditional peanut butter cups for almond butter versions, using dark chocolate and natural almond butter for a healthier alternative.

5. Chia Seed Pudding: Creamy and Nutrient-Rich

Chia seeds, when soaked in liquid, become a creamy pudding-like consistency without the need for added sugar or dairy:

a. Vanilla Chia Pudding: Mix chia seeds with almond milk and a hint of vanilla extract. Let it sit in the fridge until it thickens, and then top with fresh berries for a guilt-free dessert.

b. Chocolate Chia Pudding: Add unsweetened cocoa powder and a touch of honey to your chia seed pudding mix for a chocolatey treat.

6. Sorbet and Frozen Treats: Cool and Refreshing

Sorbet and homemade frozen treats can be a healthy and refreshing way to enjoy dessert:

a. Berry Sorbet: Puree frozen berries with a squeeze of lemon juice and a touch of honey or agave nectar. Freeze until firm for a fruity and guilt-free sorbet.

b. Frozen Yogurt Bark: Spread Greek yogurt on a baking sheet, top with sliced fruits and a drizzle of honey, and freeze until firm. Break into pieces for a delightful frozen treat.

By incorporating these guilt-free dessert options into your culinary repertoire, you can satisfy your sweet cravings while prioritizing your health and well-being. These desserts prove that you don't have to compromise on taste or your dietary goals to enjoy a delightful and wholesome treat.

Chapter 7: Maintaining Your Ornish Lifestyle

The Ornish Lifestyle, developed by Dr. Dean Ornish, is a comprehensive approach to health and well-being that focuses on making sustainable lifestyle changes to improve overall health, prevent chronic diseases, and enhance longevity. Whether you've recently adopted the Ornish Lifestyle or have been following it for some time, maintaining this holistic approach to health is key to reaping its long-term benefits. In this guide, we will explore essential strategies for sustaining the Ornish Lifestyle and enjoying a healthier, more fulfilling life.

1. Mindful Nutrition: One of the cornerstones of the Ornish Lifestyle is a plant-based diet that is low in fat and refined carbohydrates. To maintain this dietary approach, consider the following tips:

- **Meal Planning:** Plan your meals ahead of time to ensure you have access to nutritious options that align with the Ornish principles.

- **Variety:** Experiment with a wide variety of fruits, vegetables, whole grains, legumes, and plant-based proteins to keep your meals exciting and satisfying.

- **Cooking Skills:** Invest in your cooking skills to prepare delicious and healthy meals at home.

2. Regular Exercise: Physical activity plays a vital role in the Ornish Lifestyle. To stay active and motivated:

- **Set Goals:** Establish realistic fitness goals and track your progress.

- **Diversify Workouts:** Engage in different forms of exercise, such as walking, yoga, swimming, or strength training, to prevent boredom and maintain muscle mass.

- **Incorporate Movement into Daily Life:** Make small changes, like taking the stairs or walking during breaks, to increase your daily activity level.

3. Stress Management: Reducing stress is essential for overall well-being. Practice stress management techniques like:

- **Meditation:** Regular meditation or mindfulness exercises can help you manage stress and maintain emotional balance.

- **Deep Breathing:** Learn deep breathing exercises to calm your nervous system and reduce stress responses.

- **Yoga:** Yoga is not only a form of exercise but also an excellent way to promote relaxation and mental clarity.

4. Social Connection: Human connections are vital for happiness and health. To maintain your social well-being:

- **Stay Connected:** Nurture your relationships with family and friends by staying in touch, scheduling regular get-togethers, or participating in group activities.

- **Join Support Groups:** Consider joining support groups or online communities of like-minded individuals who share your commitment to the Ornish Lifestyle.

5. Adequate Sleep: Quality sleep is crucial for physical and mental recovery. To ensure restful sleep:

- **Create a Sleep Routine:** Develop a consistent bedtime routine to signal your body that it's time to wind down.
- **Limit Screen Time:** Reduce exposure to screens before bedtime, as the blue light emitted can disrupt sleep patterns.
- **Maintain a Comfortable Sleep Environment:** Ensure your bedroom is conducive to sleep by keeping it dark, quiet, and at a comfortable temperature.

6. Regular Monitoring: Periodically check in with your health metrics, such as cholesterol levels, blood pressure, and weight, to ensure you are maintaining your progress and making necessary adjustments.

7. Seek Professional Guidance: Consult with a healthcare provider or nutritionist who is knowledgeable about the Ornish Lifestyle. They can provide personalized guidance, monitor your health, and address any concerns or questions you may have.

8. Celebrate Milestones: Celebrate your successes along the way. Whether it's achieving a fitness goal, maintaining a healthy weight, or simply feeling more energized, acknowledging your achievements can motivate you to stay on track.

That maintaining the Ornish Lifestyle is not about perfection but about making consistent, sustainable choices that support your overall well-being. By embracing these principles and making them a part of your daily routine, you can enjoy the long-term benefits of improved health, increased vitality, and a higher quality of life.

Staying Committed to the Diet

The Ornish Lifestyle's dietary component is a fundamental aspect of this holistic approach to health and well-being. It centers on a plant-based, low-fat, and heart-healthy diet that has been shown to prevent and even reverse chronic diseases. Staying committed to this diet is key to reaping the full benefits of the Ornish Lifestyle. Here are some strategies to help you maintain your commitment to the Ornish diet over the long term:

1. Understand the Why: To stay committed to any dietary plan, it's essential to understand why you're doing it. Educate yourself about the science behind the Ornish diet and the potential health benefits it offers. This knowledge can serve as a powerful motivator.

2. Gradual Transition: If you're new to the Ornish Lifestyle, consider making dietary changes gradually. Gradual transitions are often more sustainable and less overwhelming. Start by incorporating more plant-based meals into your diet and gradually reducing animal products and saturated fats.

3. Stock Your Kitchen: Ensure that your pantry and refrigerator are stocked with a variety of plant-based foods that adhere to the Ornish principles. Having the right ingredients readily available makes it easier to prepare nutritious meals at home.

4. Meal Planning: Plan your meals in advance. Create a weekly meal plan that includes a variety of colorful fruits, vegetables, whole grains, legumes, and plant-based proteins. Planning helps you make healthier choices and reduces the temptation to opt for less nutritious options when you're hungry.

5. Cooking Skills: Invest time in improving your cooking skills. Learning to prepare tasty, satisfying plant-based meals can make the diet more enjoyable. Experiment with new recipes and cooking techniques to keep things interesting.

6. Mindful Eating: Practice mindful eating to savor your food and recognize when you're truly satisfied. Eating slowly and paying attention to your body's hunger and fullness cues can help prevent overeating.

7. Social Support: Share your commitment with friends and family, and encourage them to join you on your journey. Having a support system can make it easier to stick to the Ornish diet, especially when dining out or attending social gatherings.

8. Seek Out Recipe Resources: There are numerous cookbooks, websites, and apps dedicated to plant-based and low-fat cooking. Explore these resources to discover delicious recipes that align with the Ornish principles.

9. Stay Informed: Keep up to date with the latest research and developments related to the Ornish Lifestyle and plant-based nutrition. This ongoing education can reinforce your commitment and help you make informed dietary choices.

10. Embrace Flexibility: While the Ornish diet is primarily plant-based and low in fat, it allows for some flexibility. Occasionally indulging in your favorite treat or incorporating small amounts of healthy fats can help you maintain a sense of balance and prevent feelings of deprivation.

11. Track Your Progress: Keep a journal of your dietary choices, physical well-being, and any improvements in your health markers. Tracking your progress can be motivating and help you stay committed.

12. Consult a Nutritionist: If you have specific dietary concerns or health issues, consider consulting a registered dietitian or nutritionist who is familiar with the Ornish Lifestyle. They can provide personalized guidance and address any nutritional questions or challenges you encounter.

That maintaining a commitment to the Ornish diet is a journey, and it's normal to face occasional challenges. Stay patient, stay motivated, and always keep your long-term health and well-being in mind. By incorporating these strategies into your daily life, you can continue to enjoy the many benefits of the Ornish Lifestyle for years to come.

Overcoming Challenges

Committing to the Ornish Lifestyle, with its focus on a plant-based diet, regular exercise, stress management, and social support, can be immensely rewarding for your health and well-being. However, like any lifestyle change, it comes with its share of challenges. Here, we'll explore common hurdles people face when maintaining the Ornish Lifestyle and offer strategies to overcome them.

1. Social Pressure: One of the most significant challenges people encounter is social pressure to conform to mainstream dietary and lifestyle norms. Friends, family, and social events often revolve around foods that may not align with the Ornish diet. Here's how to tackle this:

 - **Communication:** Explain your commitment to the Ornish Lifestyle to your loved ones. Clear communication can help them understand and support your choices.

- **Bring Your Own Dish:** When attending gatherings, offer to bring a plant-based dish that you enjoy, ensuring you have a healthy option available.

- **Be Confident:** Be confident in your choices and politely decline foods that don't fit your lifestyle. Remember, your health is a priority.

2. Cravings and Temptations: Cravings for unhealthy foods can be challenging to overcome. Here's how to manage them:

- **Healthy Alternatives:** Identify satisfying, healthy alternatives for your cravings. For example, if you crave something sweet, opt for a piece of fruit or a small serving of dark chocolate.

- **Mindful Eating:** Practice mindful eating to savor your food and be more aware of your cravings. Often, the craving will pass if you take a moment to pause and reflect.

3. Time Constraints: Maintaining the Ornish Lifestyle can require more time for meal preparation and exercise. To overcome time constraints:

- **Meal Prep:** Dedicate time each week to meal prep. Cook in batches and freeze portions for busy days.

- **Short Workouts:** You don't need hours at the gym. Short, intense workouts or incorporating physical activity into your daily routine can be just as effective.

4. Travel and Dining Out: Traveling or dining out can be challenging when trying to stick to the Ornish Lifestyle. Here's how to navigate these situations:

- **Plan Ahead:** Research restaurants that offer plant-based options or call ahead to inquire about menu choices.

- **Pack Snacks:** Bring healthy snacks when traveling to avoid resorting to less nutritious options on the road.

- **Request Modifications:** Don't be afraid to ask for modifications to dishes when dining out. Many restaurants are accommodating to dietary requests.

5. **Plateaus and Slow Progress:** It's normal to experience plateaus in weight loss or other health improvements. To overcome these challenges:

- **Focus on Non-Scale Victories:** Look beyond the scale. Celebrate improvements in energy levels, sleep quality, and overall well-being.
- **Adjust and Experiment:** If you hit a plateau, consider making subtle adjustments to your diet or exercise routine. Experiment to find what works best for your body.

6. **Lack of Motivation:** Staying motivated long-term can be tough. Here's how to keep your motivation alive:

- **Set New Goals:** Continuously set new, achievable goals to keep your motivation high.
- **Join a Support Group:** Joining a group of like-minded individuals or seeking the guidance of a coach or therapist can provide ongoing motivation and accountability.

7. Stress and Emotional Eating: Stress and emotions can lead to unhealthy eating habits. To combat emotional eating:

- **Stress Management:** Practice stress management techniques such as deep breathing, meditation, or yoga.
- **Mindful Eating:** Be aware of emotional triggers and practice mindful eating to make conscious food choices.

8. Health Setbacks: Health setbacks or medical conditions can be discouraging. In such situations:

- **Consult a Healthcare Professional:** Seek guidance from a healthcare provider who understands the Ornish Lifestyle and can help you navigate health challenges.
- **Stay Committed to Your Goals:** Maintain your commitment to the Ornish Lifestyle, as it may support recovery and overall well-being.

Remember that setbacks and challenges are a natural part of any lifestyle change. What's important is your ability to adapt and persevere. Seek support from healthcare professionals, friends, and family, and remember that the long-term benefits of the Ornish Lifestyle are well worth the effort. By addressing challenges head-on and staying committed to your health, you can continue to thrive in your Ornish journey.

Tracking Your Progress

Tracking your progress is a crucial aspect of maintaining the Ornish Lifestyle. It allows you to stay motivated, identify areas for improvement, and celebrate your successes along the way. Whether your goal is to prevent chronic diseases, manage your weight, or simply lead a healthier life, here are some effective ways to track your progress:

1. Health Metrics:

- **Regular Check-Ups:** Schedule regular check-ups with your healthcare provider to monitor key health metrics such as blood pressure, cholesterol levels, and blood sugar. These measurements can provide valuable insights into your overall health and the impact of the Ornish Lifestyle.

- Keep a Health Journal: Maintain a journal to record your health-related data, including weight, blood pressure readings, and any changes in medication or supplements. Tracking these metrics over time can help you and your healthcare provider assess your progress.

2. Physical Fitness:

- Set Fitness Goals: Establish clear fitness goals, whether it's walking a certain number of steps each day, completing a specific yoga routine, or increasing your strength through resistance training.

- Use Fitness Apps: Utilize fitness apps and wearables to monitor your physical activity. Many of these apps can track your steps, workouts, and even heart rate, providing a comprehensive view of your progress.

- Keep a Workout Journal: Maintain a workout journal to record your exercise routines, including the type of activity, duration, and intensity. Tracking your workouts allows you to see how far you've come and make necessary adjustments.

3. Nutrition:

- Food Diary: Keep a food diary to log your daily meals and snacks. Include details like portion sizes, ingredients, and meal times. This can help you identify any patterns, such as emotional eating or certain trigger foods.

- Nutrition Tracking Apps: There are several apps available that can help you track your daily caloric intake, macronutrient distribution, and micronutrient intake. This can be especially helpful in maintaining a balanced diet.

4. Emotional Well-Being:

- **Mood Journal:** Track your emotional well-being by maintaining a mood journal. Note your feelings, stress levels, and any emotional triggers you may encounter. This can help you identify patterns and make necessary adjustments to your stress management strategies.

- **Mindfulness Practice:** If you're incorporating mindfulness or meditation into your Ornish Lifestyle, keep a record of your practice. Note the duration and frequency of your sessions and any changes in your emotional state.

5. Weight Management:

- **Regular Weigh-Ins:** Weigh yourself consistently, such as once a week at the same time of day and under the same conditions. This can help you track changes in your weight and identify trends over time.

- **Body Measurements:** In addition to weighing yourself, measure your waist, hips, and other relevant body parts. Sometimes, changes in body composition may not be reflected in weight alone.

6. Celebrate Milestones:

- **Reward Yourself:** Set up a system of rewards for reaching specific milestones. These rewards can be non-food-related, such as a spa day, a new book, or a leisure activity you enjoy.

- **Share Achievements:** Celebrate your accomplishments with friends and family who support your Ornish Lifestyle. Sharing your successes can boost your motivation and strengthen your commitment.

7. Adjust and Adapt:

- **Regularly Evaluate and Adjust:** Periodically review your progress data and assess whether you are on track to meet your goals. If you're not seeing the desired results, be open to adjusting your dietary, exercise, or stress management strategies.

- **Consult Professionals:** Seek guidance from healthcare professionals, nutritionists, or fitness trainers if you encounter challenges or need personalized advice on maintaining the Ornish Lifestyle.

Remember that progress may not always be linear, and setbacks can occur. However, tracking your progress provides valuable insights and helps you stay accountable to your goals. By monitoring your health metrics, physical fitness, nutrition, emotional well-being, and weight management, you can maintain your commitment to the Ornish Lifestyle and continue on the path to improved health and well-being.

Conclusions

The Ornish Diet Cookbook offers a compelling and evidence-based approach to achieving improved health and well-being through dietary choices. Dr. Dean Ornish's decades of research and clinical experience have culminated in a collection of recipes that not only promote heart health but also support overall wellness.

The cookbook demonstrates that a plant-based, low-fat diet can be both delicious and satisfying. By emphasizing whole, unprocessed foods, and incorporating a wide variety of fruits, vegetables, grains, and legumes, individuals following the Ornish Diet can enjoy a diverse range of flavors and cuisines while reaping the health benefits.

One of the most striking aspects of the Ornish Diet Cookbook is its potential to reverse chronic conditions such as heart disease, hypertension, and type 2 diabetes. It underscores the power of lifestyle choices, particularly diet, in preventing and even undoing the damage caused by these ailments. This approach offers hope to those seeking alternatives to medication and invasive procedures.

Moreover, the cookbook recognizes the importance of mindful eating and the connection between physical and emotional well-being. It encourages a holistic approach to health, highlighting the role of stress reduction techniques, exercise, and social support in the pursuit of optimal health.

While the Ornish Diet Cookbook's emphasis on low-fat, plant-based eating may not suit everyone's preferences or dietary needs, it undeniably offers a well-researched and effective path to better health. Its recipes are easy to follow and provide inspiration for those looking to make significant dietary changes for their well-being.

In a world where dietary choices play a crucial role in our health outcomes, the Ornish Diet Cookbook serves as a valuable resource for individuals looking to take control of their health, reduce the risk of chronic diseases, and enjoy delicious, nutritious meals. It is a testament to the idea that what we eat can be a powerful form of medicine, and it empowers readers to make positive changes in their lives.